Just
The
Essentials

Lacee J. Preciado

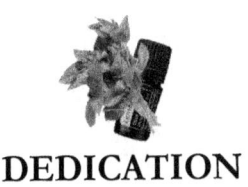

DEDICATION

To all those who have excitedly jumped on the Essential Oil train but are a little hesitant to jump off and see the sights.

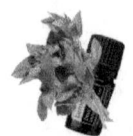

TABLE OF CONTENTS

Hi! Nice to meet you...

My name is Lacee. I have over 15 years of experience with essential oils and want to share a bit of that with you. Many people fall in love with the idea of essential oils at a class or a meet-up, order some, get home, and then think "now what." Maybe you have a sample someone gave you or you bought a diffuser. All this is great, but excitement can lead to uncertainty or even unintentional misuse. This book is designed as a reference to keep you on the right track. It is a quick uncomplicated guide to the basics of essential oils and how to use them. There are suggestions for healing along with other daily uses. I have even included portions on cooking, cleaning, scrubs...well, you'll see.

* As with all health promoting treatments, if you have any concerns or ailments, please consult a physician.

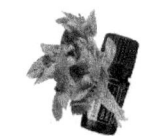

Part I: Just Try It

As you may have guessed, this is no ordinary cookbook. I'm not going to stuff it full of recipes that you will never try or fill it with information that you have no idea how to decipher. My goal is for you to be educated and inspired enough to be excited to play with your food... or face... or whatever you decide! Don't be fooled, there are some great recipes inside, but I have no doubt that you will create many more once you understand the how's and why's of using essential oils effectively in your life. This is why there are blank spaces for you to add notes and recipes of your own.

Essentials & Differences

Now, let's go over the essentials of essential oils. There are countless numbers of essential oil companies with a wide variety of... well... everything, from price to quantity to quality. Every little difference can make a difference and they all have their place.

That being said, when I consider putting something for a healthful purpose in my body, or the body of my friends and family, I tend to raise the bar a bit. This is why I choose doTERRA essential oils. Every recipe in this book was designed with doTERRA essential oils in mind. Much of the information contained in these pages, can be found in a reference guide titled <u>Modern Essentials</u> or on the doTERRA websites. This is not to say that you cannot use other brands of essential oils in these recipes, but I caution that information and quality varies from brand to brand and from oil to oil. For instance, which species of plant, where it is grown, and how it is distilled, can effect the constituents and how beneficial they are. Not all essential oils can be ingested. Some can tax your liver. Sadly when you see that little label "pure" in the store, it doesn't necessarily mean a single pure essential oil, it just means that there is not a carrier oil in it. (like coconut or jojoba)

Therefore, their health promoting qualities are not always the same even when using oils that bear the same name. This is why I always suggest researching whatever brand you choose.

doTERRA has set a new and very high bar with the testing of their oils. To assure that every batch of essential oils is perfect and pure in every way, they run a myriad of specific tests before distributing. Once the oils have passed these tests, they are marked as Certified Pure Therapeutic Grade (CPTG) Essential Oils. These CPTG essential oils are ingestible and can be used for health benefits. Every one of their essential oils have been grown indigenously and are distilled in a manner that will not alter their prized chemical compounds. Thus, you can be assured that each bottle of any given CPTG essential oil contains the exact same compounds and will continue to be effective. They are pure, they work, they are easy to get, and are sold a fair price… and for now - that is good enough for me.

Uses

Each essential oil can be used for many reasons and for many ailments. I have included a few of these ailments for each CPTG essential oil listed, as well as some precautions. It is important to keep in mind that essential oils are holistic in nature, for body, mind, and spirit. As such, they can and should be used for their body and emotional properties. For example: lavender is calming and is great for burns, peppermint can awaken the senses and soothes an upset stomach.

Administration

There are three ways to use an essential oil, aromatically, internally and topically. Just because an essential oil can be ingested, does not mean that that is the best way to take it. It is important to note that the most effective way to administer an essential oil is through aromatherapy-- smelling them directly or diffusing them in a room with a cold diffuser. As a loose rule of thumb: If the oil is needed for digestive issues, it should be ingested. If it is needed for skin issues, it should be used topically. Many can be used neat, meaning applied directly to the skin. Any thing that is placed in or on the body is absorbed and cycled throughout the entire system and finally filtered through the liver. Any application of essential oil whether used topically or ingested can penetrate every cell in the body within approximately 20 minutes. If the oil is ingested, it passes through the stomach and can be broken down by the digestive system.

There are many ways to ingest an essential oil. Many can be taken directly on the tongue or added to water. They can be placed in a capsule or even added to food. Every method has their place. That being said, if you are using essential oils for purely a health benefit... then you should do what my father would say when we were being wimps, "Just take it like a man!" To which, of course, we clever girls would respond, "and cry?" What I am trying to say is, that if you are having digestive issues, for example, you should just take the drop of needed oil directly on the tongue or in a shot of water, even if it doesn't taste pleasant. This would give you the most health value. Excessive heat and prolonged exposure to other chemicals alters the chemical make-up and reduces the health benefits. This is not to say that you cannot effectively use the oils in tea, baths, or foods. I just wouldn't boil or cook them expecting 100% of their efficacy to remain.

Portioning

As far as portioning is concerned, 1 drop of a CPTG essential oil is potent and effective. For reference, a single drop of peppermint essential oil is equivalent to over 20 cups of peppermint tea. So, when a single drop is suggested, it is wise to try only one before getting overly zealous, not to mention, their flavor is strong, so mixing well before adding more is a good idea. Like vanilla, which tastes and smells wonderful when added sparingly to a recipe, but is not very appetizing when eaten alone, essential oils need to be added carefully to a recipe. Be creative, but watch out! Just because it smells like it could complete a recipe, its taste could ruin it! Try ingredients that have a stronger taste and texture. This allows you to use the oil for their health benefits while hiding them within foods. When using for health purposes a drop or two 2-3 times a day is usually effective. For more precise portioning, use a research guide.

Essential Oils for Cooking

<u>Basil</u>

USE: migraines, respiratory and digestive problems

AFFECTS: Cardiovascular system, muscles and bones

NOTE: avoid during pregnancy, epilepsy, caution with sensitive skin

<u>Bergamot</u>

USE: fever, intestinal worms & parasites, appetite loss, insomnia, eczema, soothes lungs

AFFECTS: Digestive System, Emotional Balance, Skin

NOTE: caution with direct skin contact

<u>Cinnamon</u>

USE: stomachaches, depression, viral and infectious diseases, boosts immune system

AFFECTS: Immune System

NOTE: avoid during pregnancy, can burn nostrils and

irritate nose, caution with direct skin contact

Clove

USE: tooth pain, skin infections, antitumor

AFFECTS: Cardiovascular, Digestive, Immune, & Respiratory System

NOTE: Caution during pregnancy and with sensitive skin, caution with direct skin contact

Ginger

USE: antiseptic, digestion, flatulence, infectious disease

AFFECT: Digestive & Nervous Systems

NOTE: avoid direct sunlight for 3-6 hours after use, caution with direct & repeat skin contact

Grapefruit

USE: cancer, digestion, cellulite, water retention, lymph congestion

AFFECT: Cardiovascular System

NOTE: can be used NEAT, can replace photosensitivity causing citrus oils

Lavender

USE: UNIVERSAL oil, burns, stretch marks & scars, anxiety, lowers blood pressure

AFFECT: Cardiovascular Systems, Emotional Balance, Nervous System, Skin

NOTE: none

Lemon

USE: Neutralizer, digestive problems, food poisoning, disinfectant, fever (morning sickness)

Anti-oxidant, detoxifier

AFFECT: Digestive, Immune, & Respiratory Systems

NOTE: Avoid sunlight for up to 12 hours, can cause skin irritation with direct application

Lemongrass

USE: infectious illness, anti-inflammatory, regenerates connective tissue, digestion

AFFECT: Immune System, Muscles & Bones

NOTE: can cause skin irritation with direct application

Lime

Muscle spasms & cramps, anti-bacterial, anti-cancer

NOTE: Avoid sunlight for up to 12 hours, can cause skin irritation with direct application

Marjoram

USE: food poisoning, stiff joints, sprains, arthritis

AFFECT: Cardiovascular System, Muscles & Bones

NOTE: Caution during pregnancy

Oregano

USE: colds, asthma, balances metabolism, bronchitis

AFFECT: Immune & Respiratory Systems, Muscles & Bones

NOTE: can cause extreme skin irritation

Peppermint

USE: digestion, indigestion, hot flashes, motion sickness, nausea

AFFECT: Digestive System, Muscles & Bones, Nervous & Respiratory Systems, Skin

NOTE: can cause contact sensitization, caution with high blood pressure & pregnancy

Rosemary

USE: lowers blood pressure, diabetes, staph & strep infections, fatigue

AFFECT: Immune, Respiratory, & Nervous Systems

NOTE: Avoid with pregnancy, epilepsy, high blood pressure

Thyme

USE: antibacterial, anthrax, dermatitis, psoriasis, infectious illnesses, respiratory issues

AFFECT: Immune System, Muscles & Bones

NOTE: Avoid during pregnancy, caution with high blood pressure, may be irritating to mucus membranes

Wild Orange

USE: cardiac spasm, anxiety, colds, colic, lowers high cholesterol, obesity, tissue repair, fever, mouth ulcers, muscle soreness

AFFECT: Digestive & Immune Systems, Emotional Balance, Skin

NOTE: Avoid direct sunlight for up to 12 hours

On Guard

Blend of Wild Orange, Clove, Cinnamon Bark, Eucalyptus, Rosemary

USE: Great for boosting immune system, antibacterial, antiviral, anti-mold

NOTE: Caution during pregnancy /Caution with direct skin contact

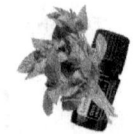

Part II: Baby Steps

Pureeing whole, fresh foods or family dinners is a great and easy way to add essential oils and other important nutrients to your child's meals.

1. Cook food
2. Puree in blender or food processor
3. Cool
4. Add 1-2 drops CPTG essential oil and serve or freeze

To freeze, spoon food into ice cube trays, cover with plastic wrap and put in freezer. Once frozen, remove "food cubes" and place in plastic freezer bags marking them with the date and type of food. Use within the month. Each cube is about one ounce.

When adding CPTG essential oils it is best to do so after foods have been cooked. Blend well and then serve.

Ideas for single items:

Vegetables - carrots, peas, squash, pumpkin, spinach, broccoli

Fruits - apricots, peaches, pears, apples, melons (freeze in chunks), bananas

Family meals:

Chicken and rice, spaghetti, mac and cheese, enchiladas, lasagna, eggplant parmesan

Don't be afraid to combine flavors, such as pumpkin and apples or carrots and pears. As for the CPTG essential oils, add one drop to enough food to make one tray according to the needs of your child.

NOTE: For those CPTG essential oils suggested for topical application below, add to a carrier oil (For example: coconut, almond or sesame oil) and then use on the skin only.

My baby has:

Baby acne - lavender (topically)

Burns – lavender (internally or topically)

Constipation - rosemary

Colic - bergamot, ylang ylang

Diaper rash - lavender (topically)

Digestion - lemon, wild orange

Eczema - helichrysum (topically)

Gas - ginger (internally & rub on belly)

Growth spurts - lemongrass

Jaundice - geranium, rosemary, lemon

Rashes - lavender, roman chamomile, melaleuca (topically with a carrier oil)

Sunburn - lavender (topically)

Teething - clove directly to gums to numb (this one is REALLY strong, but after the initial shock it is very effective)

Thrush - melaleuca, lavender

NOTE: Keep essential oils out of the eyes. It shouldn't do damage, but it can sting. You can flush with a carrier oil, like coconut - but I suggest you just avoid all that. This is why topical use on the bottom of the foot, before putting on their socks, is the safest bet.

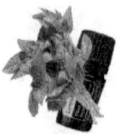

Part III: For Here or To Go?

Whether you are packing your child's lunch or sitting down to dinner, we want our family healthy and ready for anything. So why not add extra nutrients to some good ol' favorites. Remember that prolonged exposure to heat will degrade the health benefits of the essential oils.

<u>Immune Boosting Peanut Butter</u>

- 2 T peanut butter
- 1 drop cinnamon CPTG essential oil

Great for sandwiches, with fruit or on crackers

<u>Yogurt</u>

- 1 C plain or vanilla yogurt
- 1 drop lemon CPTG essential oil

Directions:
Stir well before serving

The Easiest Fruit Salad

- 1 lg can fruit cocktail, mostly drained
- 1 med can mandarin oranges, mostly drained
- 3 cups mini marshmallows
- 1 lg container cool whip
- 3 drops lemon CPTG essential oil

Directions:
1. After Cool Whip has been thawed in refrigerator overnight, add 3 drops lemon CPTG essential oil, stir well
2. In large bowl mix first 3 ingredients together with Cool Whip mixture
3. Stir well, chill before serving

Mom's Guacamole

- 4-5 avocados
- a shake or two of minced onions, dried
- a sprinkle of garlic salt
- a bit of season salt
- a dash of pepper
- a pinch of salt
- 2-3 T mild salsa
- 4 drops lemon CPTG essential oil

Directions:
1. Peel and mash avocados.
2. Add a dash of all seasonings, to taste. (sorry! That's the way that mom does it)
3. Add salsa and essential oil, stir well.

Serve with chips or spread on a warm tortilla.

Another Tasty Fruit Salad

- 1 pint sour cream
- 1 sm pkg vanilla instant pudding
- 1 C mini marshmallows
- 1 sm can pineapple chunks. drained
- 1 med can mandarin oranges, drained
- 1 C green apples, diced
- 1 C red apples, diced
- 1 lg banana, sliced
- 1 drop lime CPTG essential oil (or wild orange)

Directions:
1. In small bowl, mix sour cream, essential oil, and pudding mix
2. In large bowl toss remaining ingredients together
3. Pour mixture over fruit, stir until fully coated
4. Chill before serving

Pasta Salad

- 1 pkg spiral noodles
- 1 head of broccoli
- 1 C cubed cheddar cheese
- 1 bottle Italian dressing
- 2 drops basil CPTG essential oil

Directions:
1. Cook noodles. Drain and set aside.
2. Add basil to bottle of dressing, shake well.
3. Break up broccoli into bite size pieces.
4. Mix all ingredients together in large bowl.
5. Refrigerate. Serve cold.

Chinese Chicken Salad

Salad:

- 1 head lettuce
- 1 head purple cabbage
- 4 C cubed chicken
- 2 cans waterchestnuts
- 2 sm cans mandarin oranges
- 1/2 C sesame seeds
- 1/2 C slivered almonds
- 2 pkgs. ramen noodles (raw)

Dressing:

- 1/2 C olive oil
- 1/2 C sugar
- 1/2 C rice vinegar
- 1 t. salt
- 1/4 t. pepper
- 1 drop lemon CPTG essential oil

Directions:

1. In large bowl, mix all salad ingredients together
2. In small bowl, mix all dressing ingredients together. Stir well.
3. Pour dressing over salad and toss until evenly saturated.
4. Chill and serve.

Bruschetta

- 1 C diced tomatoes
- 1 drop Basil CPTG essential oil

Day 1 - Best if served fresh with chips, lightly toasted bread, or bread brushed with olive oil or Herb Butter (see recipe) and broil.

Day 2 - <u>Chicken Tacos</u>

- Cooked & shredded chicken breast
- corn tortillas

Top with bruchetta/salsa

Day 3 - <u>Spanish Rice</u>

- 1 T butter
- ½ - 1 C Bruchetta
- 1 C white rice
- 2 C water
- 1 t chopped fresh garlic
- 1 t minced onions, dried
- 1 t salt
- 1 t pepper

Directions:

1. Brown the rice in butter in a pan for a few minutes on med heat, stirring constantly.
2. Add water, bruchetta, rice, garlic, minced onions, salt & pepper.
3. Cover and bring to boil for 5 minute, stirring occasionally.
4. Cover and reduce heat. Simmer for 20 minutes.

Best served warm. Add salt & pepper to taste.

<u>Rosemary Chicken</u>

- 1 T extra virgin olive oil

- 1 t garlic salt
- 1 t minced onion, dried
- 1 t pepper
- 1 drop Rosemary CPTG essential oil
- 1 chicken breast

Directions:

1. Blend first 5 ingredients in small bowl.
2. Coat bottom of frying pan with the mixture.
3. Place pan over medium heat. Add chicken.
4. Flip chicken breast making sure both sides are coated with blend.
5. Cook well. Serve with rice or pasta.

Cooked Veggies

- 1 zucchini
- 1 yellow squash
- 5 white mushrooms
- 1-2 T olive oil
- 1-2 t sea salt
- 1 drop lemongrass CPTG essential oil

Directions:

1. Chop vegetables.
2. Cook in frying pan, with olive oil.
3. Add sea salt. Stir occasionally.
4. Remove from heat and stir in essential oil.
5. Serve warm.

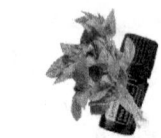

Part IV: Down Time

Whether you're wishing someone would put you in time out or you're feeling a bit run down and want a pick me up, try one of these essentials in a cup.

Note: All drinks containing CPTG essential oils are best if not kept in low grade plastic. (i.e. standard water bottles that come in a case) The oils can breakdown the low grade plastic bottles. Glass, stainless steel, ceramic, or high grade plastic is best. Remember increased exposure to high heat decreases the effectiveness of the essential oil. Essential oils are best added to hot drinks after boiling, steeping, or steaming is complete.

Flavored Water

- 8-12oz of water
- 1 drop Lemon CPTG essential oil

Directions:
Place drop of CPTG essential oil in water, and stir vigorously.

Suggestions: Lemon, Wild Orange, Lime
(also good in seltzer water)

Hot Chocolate/ Coffee

- Make your favorite hot chocolate/coffee
- Add 1 drop of the CPTG essential oil of your choice
- Stir and enjoy!

Suggestions: Peppermint, Cinnamon, Wild Orange, Clove, On Guard

Hot Tea

- 8-12oz of water
- 1 drop Peppermint CPTG essential oil
- 1 T honey (optional)

Directions:
1. Heat Water. Pour into mug.
2. Add 1 drop of the CPTG essential oil of your choice

Suggestions: Peppermint, Clove, Ginger, On Guard, Wild Orange, Lemon

Milk

- 8-12oz of milk
- 1 drop Lemon CPTG essential oil

- 1 T honey or sugar (optional)

Directions:

Serve cold.

-OR-

1. Heat milk. Pour into mug.
2. Add Lemon CPTG essential oil. Stir well.

Can substitute any essential oil you choose

Suggestions: Clove, Ginger, On Guard, Wild Orange, Peppermint

*Cinnamon is my favorite - in water with honey or in warm milk. Boost the immune system and tastes great.

*Don't forget to heat first and add oil(s) after.

Smoothies

Any ingestible CPTG essential oil can be added to a smoothie. A single drop should not alter the flavor of your smoothie very much. This is a great place to "hide" a drop. Citrus oils are a great addition for both flavor and efficacy. To assure that the CPTG essential oil is mixed in well. It is best to first blend it with a liquid.

- 1 cup orange juice
- ½ cup milk
- 1 drop lime CPTG essential oil
- 6 frozen strawberries
- 1 T almonds

Directions:
1. Blend orange juice, milk and essential oil on low for 30 seconds.

2. Add remaining ingredients and blend to desired consistency.

Suggestion: if using fresh fruit, add ice as desired

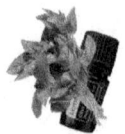

Part V: With a Cherry on Top

I know what you are probably thinking. If you are a "health-type" person you wouldn't be eating these kinds of desserts. But I say, why not split the difference. If my treat can have a health benefit inside… it's like a win/win, happy taste buds/happy body. Besides, you don't want to be the mom who sends a bowl of toasted almonds to school with your kids for the class party. Do you? ☺

Rice Krispies® Treats

- 3 T butter or margarine
- 1 10 oz package, about 40 regular marshmallows
  - OR -

- 4 cups miniature marshmallows
- 6 cups Rice Krispies®

Flavor

- 5 drops wild orange CPTG essential oil
- 2 drops clove CPTG essential oil
  - OR -
- 1 drop cinnamon CPTG essential oil

- OR -

- 2 drops grapefruit

(frost with white frosting mixed with 1 drop lemon CPTG essential oil)

Directions:

1. In large saucepan melt butter over low heat. Add marshmallows and stir until completely melted. Remove from heat.
2. Add CPTG essential oil(s). Stir completely.
3. Add Kelloggs Rice Krispies®. Coat completely.
4. Press mixture into 9 x 13 pan coated with cooking spray. Cool. Cut into 2-inch squares. Best if served the same day.

Microwave Directions:

1. In microwave-safe bowl heat butter and marshmallows on HIGH for 3 minutes, stirring after 2 minutes. Stir until smooth.
2. Follow remaining steps above. (shorten microwaving time if cutting recipe)
3. Store in airtight container. To freeze, place in airtight container, separating layer with wax paper.

Best if only kept frozen for 5 weeks. Let stand at room temperature for 15 minutes before use.

Note: Grapefruit cuts the sweetness without adding any noticeable flavor. Lemon frosting is a great topping for it. Add 1-2 drops lemon CPTG essential oil to a container of store bought white frosting, or make your own.

Fluffy Frosting

- 2 egg whites
- 1 1/2 cups sugar
- dash of salt
- 1/3 cup water
- 2 teaspoons light corn syrup
- 1 teaspoon vanilla extract
- 1 drop CPTG essential oil

Directions:

1. Combine all ingredients except vanilla in the top of a double boiler over boiling water.
2. Beat with electric mixer for about 7 minutes, or until mixture will stand in stiff peaks.
3. Beat in 1 teaspoon vanilla extract and 1 drop essential oil.

Popcorn Balls

- 3/4 cup light corn syrup
- 1/4 cup butter or margarine

- 2 t cold water
- 2 ½ cups confectioners' sugar
- 1 cup small marshmallows
- 4 cups plain popped popcorn
- 2 drops wild orange CPTG essential oil

Directions:

1. In a saucepan over medium heat, combine the first 5 ingredients. Stir continuously until the mixture comes to a boil.
2. Remove from heat.
3. Stir in essential oil
4. Slowly stir in popcorn, coating each kernel.
5. Grease hands with butter or cooking spray and quickly form the coated popcorn into balls while mixture is warm.
6. Wrap each popcorn ball with plastic wrap
7. Store at room temperature.

Orange Fudge

- 3 cups semisweet chocolate chips
- 1 (14 ounce) can sweetened condensed milk
- 1/4 cup butter or margarine
- 3-4 drops wild orange CPTG essential oil

Directions:

1. Heat on stove on low stirring occasionally
2. Once mixture has been removed from heat, add CPTG essential oil and stir well
3. Pour into well-greased 8x8-inch glass baking dish. Refrigerate until set.

Jello Cake

- 1 white cake mix with all ingredients
- 1 lg box raspberry Jello
- 1 lg container Cool Whip

Directions:
1. Bake cake as directed. Let cool.
2. Mix Jello as directed.
3. Poke hole into the top of cake with back of wooden spoon, making sure to not go deeper than half way.
4. Pour warm Jello mixture onto cake.
5. Place in refrigerator to cool.
6. Top with Cool Whip and serve.
   (see Cool Whip directions below, using lime essential oil)

Cool Whip

- 1 lg container Cool Whip
- 2 drops CPTG essential oil of your choice

Directions:
1. Let cool whip sit out for 20 min. or until soft or place in refrigerator overnight.
2. Stir in 2 drops CPTG essential oil of your choice.

Suggested oils: Lemon, Cinnamon,

Wild Orange, Lime, Clove, Peppermint

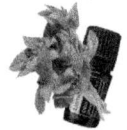

Part VI: Just A Little Extra On The Side

Dips, Sauces, Dressings, and Spreads are a fun way to use essential oils in foods. Let me remind you once again, 1 drop of CPTG essential oil is potent and a night in the refrigerator will increase its flavor.

*This area is where I like to get creative.

Carmel Dip

- 8oz cream cheese, softened
- ¾ C packed brown sugar
- 8oz sour cream
- 2 t vanilla extract
- 1 C cold milk

- 3.4oz pkg instant vanilla pudding mix
- 1 t lemon juice
- 1 drop lemon CPTG essential oil

Directions:

1. In large bowl, beat cream cheese and brown sugar until smooth
2. Add remaining ingredients one at a time, beat well after each addition
3. Cover and refrigerate
4. Serve cold with fresh fruit

Thick Italian Dressing

- 1 C yogurt
- 1 ½ T olive oil
- 1 T parmesan
- 1 t lemon juice
- 1 t garlic salt
- 1 drop basil CPTG essential oil
- 1 drop lemon CPTG essential oil

Directions:

Stir together in bowl, toss with salad

Note: Dressing will be thick

Peanut Butter Yogurt Fruit Dip

- 1 C plain yogurt
- 1 T peanut butter
- 1 drop cinnamon CPTG essential oil

Directions:

1. Mix all yogurt and essential oil, stir well.
2. Add Peanut butter and stir until fully blended

Best if served fresh & cold

Fruit Dip

- 8oz. whipped cream cheese
- 8oz marshmallow cream
- 1-2 drops lavender CPTG essential oil

Directions:

1. Mix well
2. Serve cold

Try bananas.

Tasty Veggie Dip

- 1 c. mayonnaise
- 1 ¼ C sour cream
- 1 T chopped onions, dried
- 2 t garlic salt
- 1/2 tsp. pepper
- 2 T parsley flakes, dried
- 2 T grated parmesan cheese, powdered
- 1 drop rosemary CPTG essential oil

Directions:

Combine all ingredients in bowl. Best if chilled before serving. Serve fresh.

Pita Crisps

- 1 Package of pita bead
- 2 T Wild Orange butter

Directions:

1. Cut regular sized pitas into wedges.
2. Brush with Wild Orange Butter (see recipe)
3. Oven bake at 350 degrees until crispy.

Note: For variety, brush first with oil, a little garlic powder and parmesan cheese or sprinkle on a little water, cinnamon and brown sugar. Serve with a favorite dip, yogurt or apple sauce.

Wild Orange Butter

- 2-3 T butter
- 1 drop wild orange CPTG essential oil

Mix well and enjoy!

Cinnamon Honey Butter

- 3 T butter
- 1 T honey
- 1 drop cinnamon CPTG essential oil

Mix honey and cinnamon CPTG essential oil together first, then add butter. Mix well.

Herb Butter

- ½ C butter
- 1 drop CPTG essential oil
- ½ t garlic salt

Mix well and enjoy!

Suggested oils: Basil, Oregano, Rosemary

Great on pasta, cooked chicken or steak, broiled garlic bread

Cinnamon Syrup

- 1 C sugar
- ¼ C water
- ½ C corn syrup
- 5 oz. can evaporated milk
- 1 T butter
- 1 drop cinnamon CPTG essential oil

Directions:

1. In small saucepan, combine sugar, water, and corn syrup
2. Bring to boil. Stir constantly.
3. Cook for 2 minutes.
4. Remove from heat.
5. Add milk, butter and essential oil
6. Serve warm with pancakes, french toast, or waffles

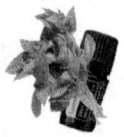

Part VII: Quick! Hide In Here

If you have an essential oil that you want to ingest, but you can't seem to stomach the flavor, look no further. These flavors are strong enough to mask most essential oils. Keep the family healthy without them knowing. For hot items, cook first, remove from heat, and then add in the oil.

*Don't forget that cooking an essential oil causes it to lose some (or all) of its health benefits. Don't worry. It is still a safe flavoring agent, but you don't want to boil it and assume it is at its best.

Spaghetti Sauce

Pizza Sauce

Cocktail Sauce

Ketchup

BBQ Sauce

Salsa

Mustard

Most Salad Dressings

Cranberry Sauce (use a citrus essential oil)

Jello (use a citrus essential oil, because let's face it…oregano Jello is just nasty!)

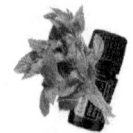

Part VIII: Slumber Parties

Are your girls having their first slumber party, are you just a little short on cash this month, or better yet... shhhh... do you just want to feel like a kid again? Well, get out the oatmeal, eggs, and honey...You'll be set to slather food on your face and proudly say it is in the name of beauty!

For direct application to skin, sometimes it is best to use a carrier oil for application. A general rule mix 2 drops CPTG essential oil with 2 T coconut oil. A patch test can be performed on the inside of forearm or behind ear to check for sensitivities.

Note: It is always wise to do a patch test behind your ear for skin allergies or sensitivities before placing any new substance on your face. Leave on for 10-20 minutes for a reaction before proceeding with the mask. If allergy or sensitivity occurs, applying Lavender CPTG essential oil directly to the affected area can help to calm the skin.

Essential Oils

Lemon

USES: Brightens complexion, removes dead skin cells.

NOTE: Caution with direct sunlight for 12 hours after use. Can irritate skin

Frankincense

USES: Anticancer, anti-inflammatory, antitumor, prevents scarring, decreases wrinkles

Helps improve focus and meditation, decreases hyperactivity

Geranium

USES: Antibacterial, antiseptic, heavy menstrual flow, tumors, acne, eczema, ringworm, oily skin, cleanser

NOTE: Can cause contact sensitization with repeat use, can be used NEAT

Peppermint

USES: Headaches, arthritis, depression, radiation exposure, soothes & cools skin

NOTE: Can cause contact sensitization with repeat use

Melaleuca (a.k.a. Tea Tree)

USES: Antiviral, antibacterial, antifungal - keeps skin clean

NOTE: Can cause contact sensitization with repeat use. Dilute with carrier oil

Myrrh

USES: Cancer, herpes, viral hepatitis, eczema, decongests prostate gland, ringworm, inflamed or chapped skin, wrinkles

NOTE: Caution during pregnancy

Lavender

USES: Good for dehydrated skin, wrinkles, and stretch marks, burns, inflammation, sunburns, lymphatic drainage

Helichrysum

USES: Good for eczema, helps reduce scarring, stops bleeding, reduces hematomas, stimulates liver cell function, regenerates tissue, varicose veins

Roman Chamomile

USES: Cleanses liver & aids it rejecting poison, acne, boils, sensitive skin, reduces irritability, soothes fever, aids nervousness, good for shock

NOTE: Dilute for those with sensitive skin, can irritate

Ylang Ylang

USES: Helps regulate blood pressure, great as a hair tonic (split ends), anxiety, balances equilibrium, increases sexual energy, helps stimulate immune system

NOTE: Can cause contact sensitization with repeat use

Masks & Scrubs

Simple Essential Oil Blend

Mix 1/2 T coconut oil with 1-2 drops of the CPTG essential

oil of your choice.

Apply to whole of face, gently rub into skin

Oatmeal Mask - For troubled skin

Mix together oatmeal and water to form a paste. Add 2-3 drops of the CPTG essential oil of your choice. Apply to face and leave on for 9 minutes.

Rinse off with warm water, finish with a rinse of cool water and enjoy soft, exfoliated skin.

Oatmeal Egg Mask- For normal/combo skin

Mix 1 egg, ½ cup cooked instant oatmeal, and a teaspoon of olive oil together with 2 drops of the CPTG essential oil of your choice. Stir until smooth.

Dampen face with warm moist cloth.

Spread mixture on face and let sit for 15 minutes.

Rinse with cool water. Towel dry.

Egg Yolk Mask - For dry skin

Mix 2-3 raw egg yolks together with 2 drops of the CPTG essential oil of your choice.

Dampen face with warm moist cloth.

Spread mixture on face and let sit for 15 minutes.

Rinse with cool water.

Towel dry.

<u>Egg Yolk & Honey Mask</u> - For dry skin

Mix 2 raw egg yolks, ½ T olive oil, and 1 T honey together with 2 drops of the CPTG essential oil of your choice.

Dampen face with warm moist cloth.

Spread mixture on face and let sit for 10-20 minutes.

Rinse with warm water.

Splash cold water upon face before drying with towel.

<u>Egg Whites Mask</u> - For oily skin

Mix 2-3 raw egg whites together with 2 drops of the CPTG essential oil of your choice.

Dampen face with warm moist cloth.

Spread mixture on face and let sit for 15 minutes.

Rinse with cool water.

Towel dry.

<u>Carrot Mask</u> - For oily skin

Blend cooked carrots then take ½ cup and stir in 2-3 drops of the CPTG essential oil of your choice.

Dampen face with warm moist cloth.

Spread mixture on face and let sit for 10 minutes.

Rinse with cool water.

Towel dry.

(this will make you appear a bit tan)

Honey Mask

Mix 3 T Honey with 2-3 drops of the CPTG essential oil of your choice.

Dampen face with warm moist cloth.

Spread mixture on face and let sit for 10-20 minutes.

Rinse with warm water.

Splash cold water upon face before drying with towel.

Black Head Remover

Mix 2 raw egg whites and 3 drops of lemon juice together with 2 drops of the CPTG essential oil of your choice.

Dampen face with warm moist cloth.

Spread mixture on face and let sit for 10-20 minutes.

Rinse with cool water.

Towel dry.

Brown Sugar Body Scrub

Mix 1 cup brown sugar, 2-3 T of coconut oil, and 1-2 drops of the CPTG essential oil of your choice.

Scrub body to exfoliate.

Rinse with warm water.

Salt Body Scrub

Mix 1 T kosher salt, 2-3 T of olive oil, and 1-2 drops of the CPTG essential oil of your choice.

Scrub rough areas (especially heals and elbows) to exfoliate. Avoid eyes.

Rinse with warm water.

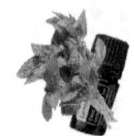

Part IX: Spring Cleaning

It's that time of the year again. Nobody likes having to clean, but we all love the results. Well, this time, your home will be sparkling, there will be no lingering dangerous chemicals, and the air will smell great with whichever essential oil you choose.

Using CPTG essential oil in place of standard household cleaning products can reduce the amount of toxins released into the air by the cleaning products. Of the tens of thousands of chemicals used commercially today, over 90% of them are considered hazardous to our health.

Essential oils are anti-viral, anti-fungal, anti-bacterial, don't leave a toxic residue, and are therefore safe for children and pets. The fragrance left behind can be uplifting and health promoting for those exposed to it. And if your bottle of cleaning products is accidently ingested by your little ones, they won't have to be rushed to the emergency room.

Cleaning with CPTG essential oils is safe and easy. Just fill a spray bottle with water, add 5-10 drops of the essential oil of choice, shake, and use. This can also be used in cars, playpens, tents, cleats, gym bags...

Diffusing CPTG essential oils in the air can neutralize the air and kill virus, bacteria, and fungus. This can and should be done in any room in the house. Think kitchens, bathrooms, and even children's bedrooms and playrooms.

NOTE: some oils are strong and diffusing them can irritate the eyes and mucous membranes of the nose.

Ex. Oregano, Cinnamon

CPTG essential oils can also be used neat. (Neat=direct application) Drop directly into the toilet bowl between cleanings.

Suggested Oils for Cleaning

Citrus Bliss

A blend of citrus oils including: lemon, grapefruit, wild orange, bergamot, mandarin, tangerine, and clementine with a bit of vanilla. This blend is uplifting to the mood and a powerful disinfectant.

Lemon

Lemon is a great neutralizer, for both the body and the environment. It can be safely used internally, topically, and aromatically. It is non-toxic so it perfect for all surfaces of the home and works well in a variety of setting. Diffusing it in a home or office is a great way to purify the air, and like most citrus oils it is uplifting to the mood. (This is one of my favorite oils for its versatility and effectiveness, not to mention its low price point.)

Melaleuca

Also known by the name Tea Tree. It is most commonly known for being a powerful anti-viral, anti-fungal, and anti-bacterial oil. It is great for cleansing surfaces as well as the skin. (This is another favorite of mine for cleaning.)

On Guard

Is a blend that is immune boosting and a powerful fighter of pathogens, viruses, illnesses. It can be diffused, or used directly to clean and purify.

Purify

It contains lime, lemon, citronella, pine, cilantro, and melaleuca. This blend of many citrus oils can eliminate strong odors and contaminates. It is said to be able to neutralize the odor of a can of paint when added. It can purify surfaces, air, and the body. (Use aromatically and topically only)

Wild Orange

Is great for mood enhancement. It energizes and uplifts. It can be used for cleaning with its common citrus properties. Probably best when combines with Lemon.

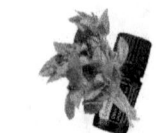

Part X: Oops A Daisy!

For all of those "oops a daisies" that happen when you are on the run. These are the few essential oils to have on hand. Carry them in your purse, your car, your backpack - and you'll be ready for most anything.

Lavender - The universal oil, cuts, scrapes, bug bites, burns, it soothes & is calming

NOTE: safe for children, pets, pregnant & nursing women

Lemon - The neutralizer - odor fighting, add in water to purify

Peppermint - Tummy soother & energizer

NOTE: can keep a little one awake so think that through if it is nap time

On Guard - Immune booster and strong anti-viral, use to sanitize hands

NOTE: I take this one orally when entering a hospital or when in contact with someone who is sick - then I use it topically after contact

ABOUT THE AUTHOR

I am a massage therapist and have been for about fifteen years, before essential oils were popular. I was introduced to essential oils then and have since taken over 100 class hours of classes on the subject. I have used them since my first class all those years ago and have continued to research and use these life-changing tools. I didn't start by using doTerra back then. The oils I began with were medical grade and amazing. I switched to the doTerra brand when I moved to a new state and had a difficult time getting the brand I respected. It is easier to discuss a single brand when suggesting the ingestion of essential oils. If you like other brands just make sure they are safe to ingest.

As an aside: I in no way think I am an expert. Save that title for those certified Aromatherapists who have taken the time to achieve that sacred title. However, I am versed enough to help get you started. I am currently a Middle School Teacher with an M.A. in Creative Writing who massages, teaches massage, and instructs on essential oils.

My hope is you that find these tools helpful, healthful, and fun.